No to belly fat

Kill the fat

Your perfect way to the dream body

You have to want it, you have to do it, no one can do it for you!

Welcome to your new life. Today is the day when I will help to become a completely new person with the help of my knowledge acquired over the years as a nutritionist.

Before we even begin with the subject, which is so difficult to implement, as so often feared, I would like to tell you here and now, the most important of all this.

Many people have excuses. A healthy lifestyle requires so much time and you have to give up everything, in addition to a lack of cooking skills, the environment, and then I have to exercise several times a week, track calories, not consume sugar, no longer with friends in restaurants eat, and so on...

People who have these thoughts are really sorry. If you just thought that, or something like that, oje.

Please do not misunderstand me. I just can't understand it. Even if a balanced diet is so important to you, and you are considering all these things above, because at last something needs to be changed about the current lifestyle and possibly your body.

Stop!

It doesn't make sense to restrict yourself so hard, it doesn't make you thinner faster, it just makes you depressed. I know what I'm talking about, I was at that stage myself.

But over the years you learn to do it, and now you can live as I want. Do you want that too?

Well then, let's start with this book, which brings you closer to your goals and gives you an insight into a healthy lifestyle.

Energy- Everything is built on

Hey, why energy now, is this about food? yes, right. That's what's in the food. If we ignore health-promoting substances, vitamins and minerals for a moment, then our food is basically only made up of energy. This energy is called kilocalories. A kilocalorie is the amount of energy needed to heat a litre of water by half a degree Celsius. This does not sound like much, but this low level of energy has an enormously important position, especially in nutrition and weight loss.

Our body needs this energy:

We need energy all the time. Whether we are sitting, walking, sleeping, our bodies constantly burn energy in the form of kilocalories.

These kcal are needed by our organism to keep the vital functions alive. These processes, which are constantly running in the body, which keep us alive, are roughly called metabolism.

So, to keep our required metabolism running, do we need what?

Proper energy in the form of calories or kilocalories. The problem is that, as the world's obesity statistics show, we seem to be taking too much of these often wrongly declared "evil" calories.

One actually thinks (if you do not deal fully with the subject) when eating food in relation to the often-large numbers of calories in which it is often incurred:

A pizza here, a beer there. As a coronation, there is a pack of chips in the evening in front of the TV, and of course a delicious white bread with butter and jam the next morning. Sounds actually very tasty, but is usually neglected,

All of this has calories, and if, like most people in the world, you are not very active, and are more likely to spend the day sitting down, then unfortunately that is too much of a *good*thing.

With a calorie surplus, i.e. too high intake of energy, the body then thinks almost the following:

Hey, you lazy human beings, what's the point? I have enough energy for today!

I hope that was explained in an easy way. Due to too much energy, signals are sent out in the body, which then make it clear to the organism that too many calories have been absorbed.

What the human body cannot need, it cancels. It then stores the excess energy as fat. Preferred and scientifically proven, this is the known annoying hip gold in the abdominal area.

Unfortunately, this hip gold does not disappear overnight. But don't worry, because we don't get fat overnight because we eat and drink too much.

This is done over a longer period of time. If it has already happened, it takes longer to get rid of the hip gold, as the body chooses itself which fat reserves it restores or reduces in the event of an energy deficiency, i.e. a calorie deficit. Targeting to burn fat is not possible.

Statements like: You can burn fat on your stomach! Abdominal exercises melt the belly fat, and even bring out a washboard belly!

... are nothing but hot air.

Calorie deficit

The magic word for constant weight loss. But beware! Don't do stupid things like 99% of all other people who want to lose weight.

We know that the body logically decompose its own reserves in the event of a lack of energy, i.e. too little energy intake.

Moment, own reserves! That doesn't just mean fat!

Driving an extreme calorie deficit over a longer period of time, i.e. radically eating much less than is needed, tends to be detrimental to weight loss as a result.

Because the body, which is in a lack of energy, initially reduces proteins in the event of a calorie deficit.

So, with a reduced energy intake, make sure that you have a sufficient protein intake!

According to experts we recommended an amount of 0.8g/kilogram body weight. If you exercise, more protein must be added (approx. 1.6g/kilogram body weight) to prevent possible muscle loss. Especially in the case of physically demanding, muscle-stressing activity, for example during strength training, where your muscles are irritated, sufficient protein must be supplied in order to maintain the trained muscles safely. Because muscles are great. Not only do you look good for many and strengthen the body, as well as make you less prone to wear and tear, or similar, they constantly burn energy. Even when we don't move, muscle cells burn calories. If you carry increased fat-free mass, i.e. muscles, with you, you can eat more because you consume more. The basic turnover is higher.

Protein

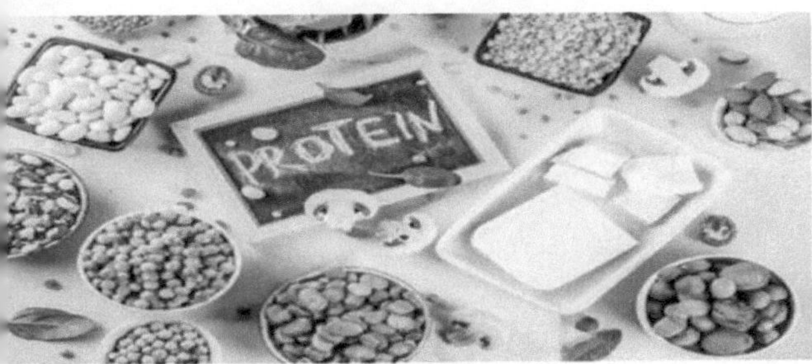

Protein - the building blocks of our body

Also called proteins are our building materials. They are components of each cell. They are made of amino acids (AS). There are 20 different ones. Of these 20 AS occurring in nature, 8 (in infants 9) are essential. This means that they must be absorbed by food, as the body cannot produce them itself. These essential amino acids are:

Isoleucine

Leucine

Lysine

Methionine

Phenylalanine

Threonine

Tryptophan

Valine

Histidine (in infants)

<u>1g protein delivers 4kcal</u>

A maximum of 15% of daily energy should be absorbed in the form of protein.

Of these, about 1/3 should come from animal origin, since animal products usually absorb saturated fats, purines and cholesterol at the same time.

Especially red meat consumption should be minimized accordingly.

Vegetable protein sources, on the other hand, provide health-rich substances such as water- and fat-soluble vitamins, minerals, fibre and phytochemicals. Therefore, the remaining 2/3 of the ingested proteins should be of plant origin.

Good protein suppliers are:

Lean fish and meats, milk and dairy products, legumes, nuts

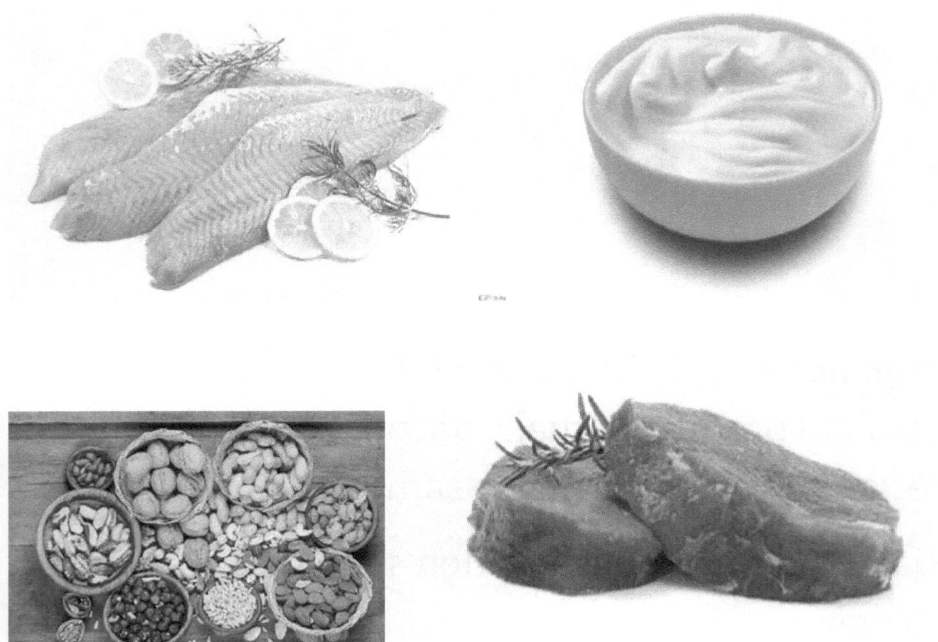

If your diet adheres to the above-declared values, a protein deficiency is very unlikely.

Protein deficiency

However, a protein deficiency is nevertheless a common and often underestimated deficiency. A lack of the important nutrient protein can have various causes and is noticeable by different symptoms. However, a wrong diet is not the only reason that protein shortages are not the only reason. Many diseases can also promote an emerging protein deficiency. The consequences for human health are sometimes very dangerous. The protein deficiency is a not to be underestimated phenomenon and, in many cases, requires medical treatment. If the organism does not get enough protein through the daily diet, it gets the necessary proteins from the muscles. One of the consequences of a protein deficiency is, of course, the breakdown of muscle mass. This leads to a slow-moving muscle weakness, which can also affect the heart muscle in the end.

Proteins are essential in life, which means essential and significantly involved in the healing of wounds. A protein deficiency leads to wound healing disorders. Hair loss and water accumulation in the tissue are other health disorders that can occur in case of a lack of protein. Especially health-conscious people who eat vegan or vegetarian should be careful not to have a protein undersupply. In addition to physical limitations, the existing deficiency also causes mental disorders. Too little high-quality protein puts stress on both the body and the soul.

As mentioned above, a lack of vital protein can have serious consequences. The causes of a protein deficiency are usually manifold. Certain diseases such as zölliakie, native sprue or existing thyroid diseases, as well as an inadequate diet or an enzyme deficiency, can lead to a protein shortage.

A protein deficiency first affects the so-called albumins. These proteins provide the necessary pressure in the cells. Albumins are responsible for 80 percent of the pressure in the circulation. A lack of protein causes the pressure to automatically decrease and water build up in the tissue. If the protein deficiency is severe or prolonged, there is therefore a risk of death. The most common cause of protein deficiency is a low protein intake through the diet. Protein deficiency can also occur as a symptom of diseases of the liver, kidney, heart or skin. In this case, the primary disease prevents the absorption of protein. An already damaged liver tissue is no longer able to produce sufficient amounts of protein. Certain hereditary diseases can also lead to a lack of protein in the body in the long term.

The deficiency can occur at any age and affects both men, women and children. Children and adolescents in the growth phase, pregnant women, the elderly and, above all, strength athletes have a particularly high protein requirement. Athletes need more protein than people who do not exercise much. The average protein requirement is about 0.8 to 1 gram per kilogram of body weight. At a size of 1.70 meters, 70 grams of protein should therefore be ingested daily with the diet. In sports such as strength training, the need for protein is much higher. For this reason, strength athletes are advised to eat 2 grams of protein per kilogram of body weight. The protein requirement increases even with hard physical work.

Typical symptoms of protein deficiency

Over a short period of time, the organism can compensate for the lack of proteins before attacking the physical reserves. The first signs of deficiency include symptoms such as hair loss, eye edges, premature wrinkle formation and weight loss. If the deficiency is not rectified immediately, muscle weakness and a reduction in muscle mass will occur. Long-term protein deficiency leads to significant health impairments. If you don't see any improvement in performance or even a drop-in performance despite daily workouts in the gym, you should check your protein supply. Loss of muscle mass could be behind the performance drop. A protein deficiency is also noticeable psychologically. Fatigue, mental and mental exhaustion, poor mood and increased sensitivity are signs of reduced mental strength. The reason for this is protein deficiency. Indigestion such as bloating and diarrhea are unpleasant and can occur if you do not drink certain foods. However, digestive problems often also indicate a deficit of protein.

Infants and children who receive too little protein often suffer from growth and thriving disorders. Increased cholesterol levels and anaemia are also symptoms that can occur with a protein deficiency. Since a protein deficiency can also indicate a serious illness, you should go to the doctor when the first symptoms appear. The diagnosis is made by means of a blood test. In order to rule out the possibility that a serious illness is the cause of the protein deficiency, your GP will carry out further examinations. If the protein deficiency is not treated in time, there is a gradual degradation of important bodily functions. Without treatment, serious complications must be expected in the case of advanced protein deficiency. Collapsed cheeks and protruding bones are clearly visible signs of a lack of proteins. At the latest, if you notice these symptoms, you should increase your protein intake and see a doctor. In case of prolonged undersupply, there is inevitably a sharp reduction in muscle mass. The lack of protein results in muscle weakness, which in turn can lead to reduced mobility. If the protein deficiency is not treated, the circulatory breakdown and the end death of the patient can occur. If you suspect a protein deficiency, you should seek medical treatment as soon as possible. In order to prevent this from getting this far, it makes sense to check the protein supply and, if necessary, supplement it with predominantly vegetable protein (due to lower pollution).

Animal proteins have a reputation for being higher quality. In this assessment, the essential amino acids are in the foreground. They are contained in animal proteins in significantly higher concentrations. However, for people who are susceptible to gout, there is a risk that this will be triggered by the intake of animal proteins. This results from the fact that animal proteins also have a higher purine, fat and cholesterol content. Those who rely on plant-based foods are increasingly absorbed by fibre, phytochemicals and slowly metabolizing carbohydrates.

It is better to keep this in mind and rely on a higher-percentage protein consumption from plant sources.

Losing weight with the help of protein

Unlike our other main nutrients, or fats and carbohydrates, protein promotes the production of the body's own proteins. These can then be used, for example, for metabolic enzymes and muscle cells. For this reason, storing protein as body fat is unlikely.

Protein is used by the body for different removal and conversion processes. This requires energy, which is provided as part of fat burning. About 25 percent of the calories ingested as protein are released as heat by so-called thermogenesis. This reduces the amount of energy in the proteins, which in turn means that a fraction of the calorie content in our food is released by the body as energy that it cannot use. By intake of protein, hormones are produced that produce peptides, which trigger an earlier feeling of satiety. Therefore, in theory it is possible to lose weight faster and consistently with an increased amount of protein.

As great as that may sound. Once again, I would warn against feeding too much protein. It makes sense to eat an increased amount of protein as an evening meal, a few hours before going to bed.

If you train hard and want to build your muscles, you should not forget that sport is only a component for perfect muscle growth. In addition to training, a proper high-protein diet is an inevitable prerequisite for success. We'll show you what really matters.

When your muscles are properly powered during exercise, they send out a signal. They demand to get stronger. In order to thicken the individual muscle fibers, they also need more energy and the right building material. Since muscles are largely made of protein, protein must also be supplied in sufficient quantity and quality for further muscle growth.

Since the intake of protein and muscle building are directly related, you should always pay attention to a sufficient protein supply. The German Society for Nutrition recommends taking 0.8 grams of protein per kilogram of body weight. For a man weighing 80 kilograms, this would be equivalent to 64 grams of protein. However, this guideline does not apply to athletes who want to build their muscles in a targeted manner, but only serves to maintain the muscles. According to experts, those who want to increase muscle mass explicitly should increase the amount to about 1.6 to 2 grams per kilogram of body weight in the start-up phase. Especially with beginners, muscles grow very fast. At this stage, the motto "a lot helps a lot" really applies. Later, 1.2 to 1.7 grams are sufficient.

It used to be assumed that there is a short time to absorb protein after the workout, which is optimal – the so-called anabolic window. According to the latest findings, a targeted protein boost is no longer necessary immediately after the workout, but can speed up storage. Other studies show that muscle building doesn't really begin until about six to eight hours after exercise. Consequently, protein should also be available at this time. It is therefore ideal to gradually pick up protein after the workout. Every two hours a portion of protein and your muscles are supplied.

What protein for muscle growth?

Time and again, protein powders or corresponding bars are not recommended. On the one hand, they are incredibly expensive in proportion, and on the other hand, they are often unnecessarily sugared. But even if you resort to good protein supplements, they are still expensive and don't bring more than a reasonable diet.

Anyone who tries to cover their protein balance with high-quality meat and fish will also be asked very clearly to pay. Other studies also show that vegetable protein should be even better than animal protein.

High performance and ideal muscle growth are also vegan, so without animal protein sources are possible. Vegetable protein sources usually have fewer calories, so your hard-trained muscles are also clearly visible at the end and not obscured by an unsightly layer of fat. Soy/tofu, quinoa or legumes such as lentils, beans and peas are particularly suitable as vegan sources of protein.

Protein and muscle building are a philosophy in itself that everyone handles differently. Those who eat a healthy and varied diet, however, usually already absorb sufficient amounts of protein with them through their normal diet. At the very least, according to research, you can safely do without dietary supplements.

Proteins or amino acids also play a very important role in our immune system. A sufficient supply of protein strengthens the immune system and therefore helps with a faster recovery, in case of occurring diseases.

<u>Also interesting to mention is the biological value (BW) of protein:</u>

The biological value indicates how many grams of body protein can be built up from 100g of food protein. Crucially, the essential AS are present in the ratio in which the body needs them. The limited limiting AS determines the BW of a food protein. Once the limiting amino acid has been consumed, the body can no longer synthesize protein from the food protein. The biological value is based on a chicken egg, to which "the highest" BW of 100 is assigned. I will explain why quotation marks are here in the next section. Again, for illustrative purposes:

E.g.: Milk has a biological value of 91. This means that the body can build up 91g of body protein from 100g of milk protein.

But now comes the highlight. In addition to the biological value, there is also the supplementary value.

This means that certain foods in combination allow the body to produce even more protein than the chicken egg.

These food combinations can be found in the following table

Combinations	Value
Whole egg 35% and potato 65%	137
Milk 75% and wheat flour 25%	123
Whole egg 60% and soy 40%	122
Whole egg 68% and wheat 25%	118
Whole egg 88% and corn 12%	114
Beans 52% and corn 48%	99
Gelatin 18% and beef 82%	98

Let us now move on to the next main nutrient, which tends to take a bad position in our diet.

We are talking about

fat

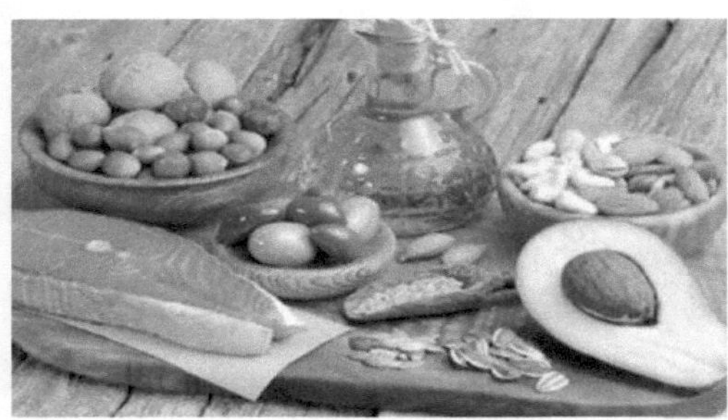 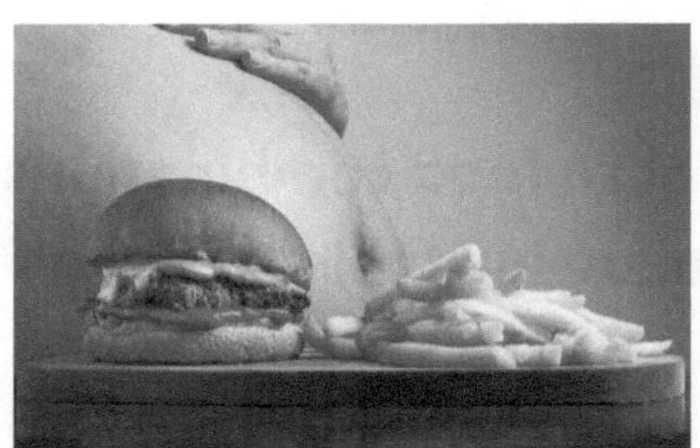

Fat is the main nutrient with the most calories and yet cannot be imagined from the diet

Fats, also called triglycerides, are compounds consisting of a glycerol molecule and three fatty acids. They are organic acids consisting of a chain of carbon atoms and a carboxyl group. They are the most energy-rich nutrient.

1g fat delivers 9kcal

High-fat foods include:

Food	Fat content/100g
Chocolate	35
Salmon	12
Bacon	40
Margarine	80
Butter	80
Oil	100
Avocado	15
Mascarpone	40
Macadamia nuts	80

There are foods where we can see the fat and which ones where we just can't see it. These fats are declared as hidden fats. According to studies, we absorb most fat in the form of hidden fats.

But fat is not the same as fat. After reading the next paragraph, you will be clear about what I mean by that.

We distinguish the fatty acids (FS) according to chain lengths:

Short-chain fatty acids, e.g. butyric acid (4:0)

Medium chain FS

6-10 Carbon Atoms

These include: capronic acid, caprylic acid and capric acid

Long-chain FS

12-24 Carbon atoms

These include: lauric acid (12:0), stearic acid (18:0)

For the numbers in parentheses, the first digit represents the number of carbon atoms and the second represents the number of double bonds contained in the compound.

However, the different fatty acids are now also classified according to the respective number of double bonds.

Saturated Fatty Acids

- You do not have double bond (DB)

- This includes e.g. stearic acid (18:0)

- Occurrences in predominantly animal foods

- They are reactive, and therefore long-lasting

- Butterfat, beef tallow, pork lard, ...

- You should make up a maximum of 10% of the total amount of fat supplied

Unsaturated fatty acids

-Own one or more Db

-This includes e.g. oleic acid (18:1)

-Occurrence mainly in vegetable foods, e.g. olive oil (69%)

-they are responsive, and therefore not long-lasting

-You should make up the majority of the fatty acid pattern at 20%

Polyunsaturated fatty acids - the essential FS

Twice unsaturated FS (€6)

-e.g. linoleic acid (18:2)

-Occurrence stake in sunflower oil (63%)

Triple unsaturated FS (s3)

e.g. a-linolenic acid (18:3)

Occurrence setherins in flax oil, flaxseeds, chia seeds, walnuts

In addition, a healthy ratio should be attached to the fatty acids

According to the guideline values of the DGE:

Omega 3: Omega 6 maximum 1:5

You need to know that fats in the diet are quite justified.

They perform important tasks in the body:

Depot grease (white fat) - protects against cold, shock and pressure

-Fat for heat regulation (brown fat)

-Fats provide fat-soluble vitamins (A, D, E, K)

-Are energy suppliers

-building blocks for the formation of hormones

Oleic acid

-No essential FS

-It lowers LDL without lowering HDL

-Protects cells from oxidative damage

Reduces the risk of cardiovascular disease and atherosclerosis

Omega-6-FS (linoleic acid, gamma-linolenic acid, arachidonic acid)

Required for:

-Wound healing

-Construction of cell membranes

-healthy growth

-Infection defense

Linoleic acid is essential

It lowers LDL but also HDL

Linoleic acid is converted to arachidonic acid (AA)

Arachidonic acid in turn is broken down into prostaglandins

They have an anti-inflammatory effect, watch out for inflammatory rheumatism

Arachidonic acid

-is formed from linoleic acid

-Occurrence only in animal fats

-Starting material for tissue hormones (prostaglandins)

-these promote rheumatic joint inflammation

However, AA is also

-vital component of cell membranes

-important for controlled duct ingenuation and skin function

-decisive for the control of gastric juice secretion

Omega-3-FS (Alpha-Linolenic Acid, EPA, DHA)

Linolenic acid is essential

-it lowers the triglyceride level in the blood

-has an antihypertensive effect

-reduces the risk of thrombosis

EPA (=eicosapenaeic acid)

-Occurrences in herring, mackerel, salmon, tuna

-is the counterparty to arachidonic acid

-anti-inflammatory, anticoagulant and vasodilator

DHA (=docosahexaenoic acid)

-Occurrence in fatty fish, see above

-important component of the retina

-protects the brain

-improves brain performance

- is part of the nerve tissue

Omega-3-FS; EPA + DHA

-are important components of the body cells

-possibly prevent depression

-Protect against cardiovascular diseases (HKK)

-strengthen the immune system

-are important for the formation of tissue hormones

Also worth mentioning are the harmful trans fatty acids (TFS)

Fortunately, these are not outstanding in the way of life of German society. However, these should not be underestimated as they have been shown to have carcinogenic properties.

TFS are created in the rumens of ruminants,

may be in some fast food products and ready meals.

Formation in the partial hydrogenation chem. Fat hardening

-heating of fats and oils at over 200°C

-TFS formation can also occur when deodorizing edible oils

A diet rich in trans fatty acids increases the concentration of LDL cholesterol in the blood and lowers that of HDL cholesterol compared to a diet rich in monounsaturated and polyunsaturated fatty acids. In addition to the cholesterol concentration in the blood, the risk of serious diseases that mainly affect the heart becomes higher.

They lower good HDL cholesterol and increase poor LDL

This increases the risk of atherosclerosis and heart disease.

Trans fatty acids can cause coronary heart disease

Important: On the ingredient lists of products they are declared as "partially hardened fats".

Ensure the lowest possible intake of these fatty acids.

Good fat sources are:

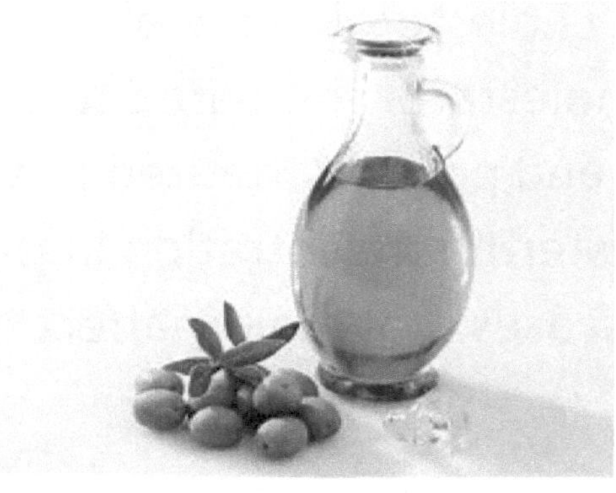

Olive oil and olives contain oleic acid, which has a positive effect on the organism

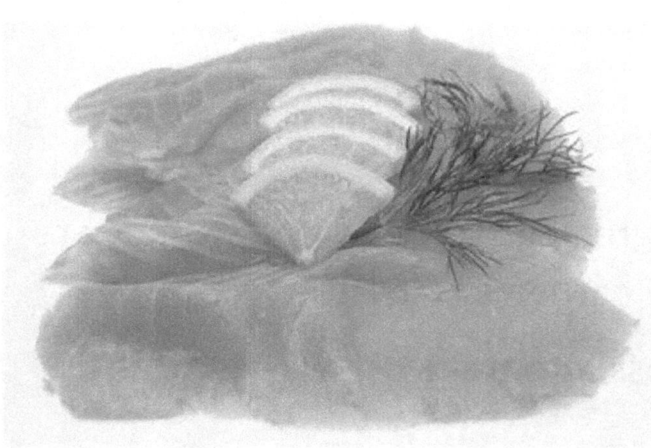

fatty sea fish (e.g. salmon)

are rich in omega-3 fatty acids

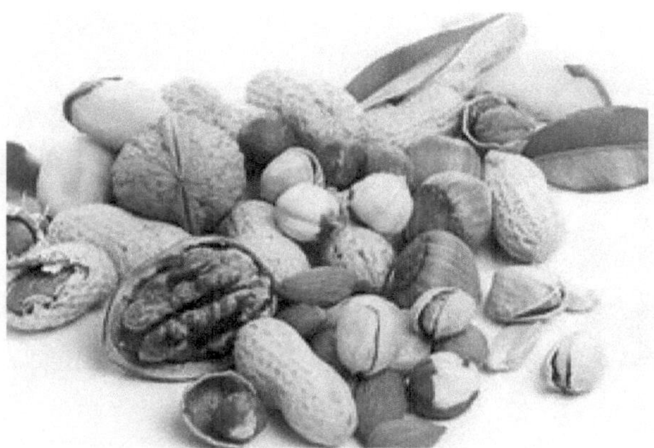

Nuts and peanuts are rich in unsaturated and polyunsaturated fatty acids. They also contain valuable minerals and vitamins

In addition to the healthy and good fat sources, there are also less suitable fat sources, and foods that contain rather unfavorable fats.

Unsuitable fats are

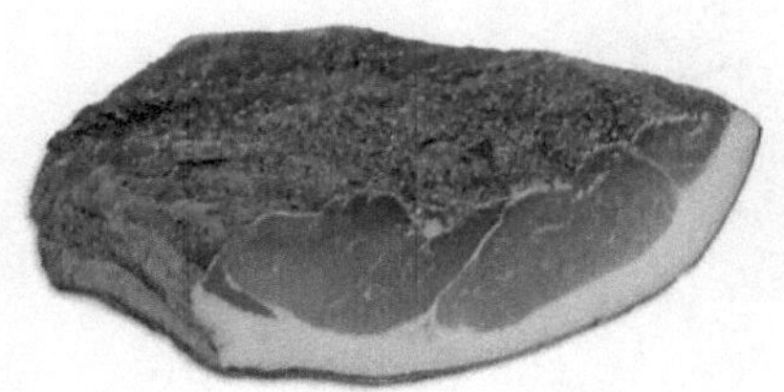

red fat meat is rich in saturated fat, and purines

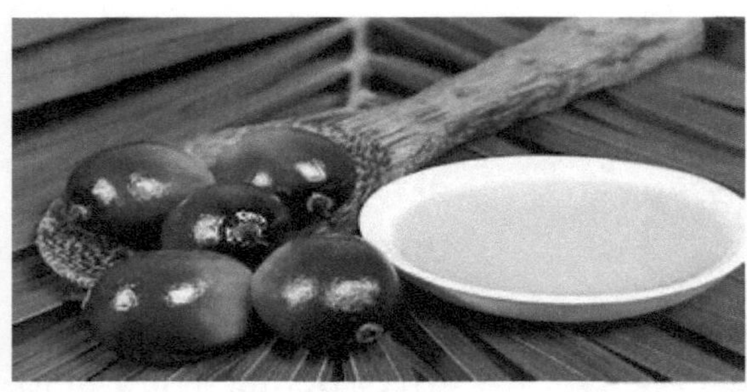

Palm fat, and sunflower oil also have an unfavorable fatty acid pattern

Especially in terms of the ratio between Omega 3 and Omega 6 FS

Carbohydrates - our main source of energy

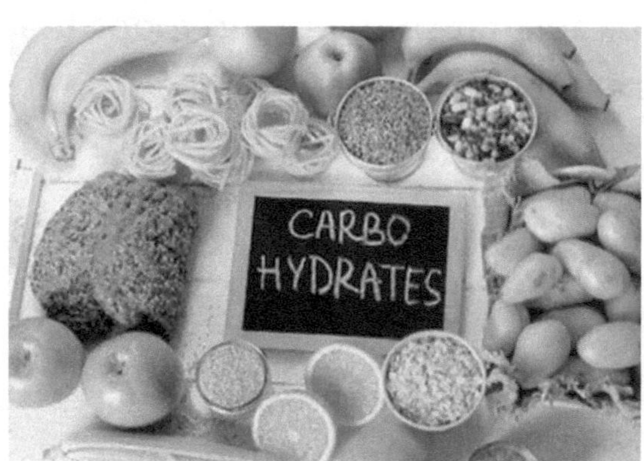

Carbohydrates are produced by photosynthesis in plants

With the help of sunlight, leafy greens (chlorophylls), carbon dioxide, and water, the plant builds up the single sugar (glucose). At the same time, it releases the essential oxygen. This is called photosynthesis.

Carbohydrates consist of carbon, hydrogen and oxygen. Together with proteins and fats, they are among the basic nutrients and are mainly found in plant-based foods.

Carbohydrates are distinguished in single sugar, double sugar and multiple sugar. Single sugar or short-chain carbohydrates are carbohydrates whose molecule contains three to seven carbon atoms.

Carbohydrates provide the body with energy:

One of the most important functions of carbohydrates is to provide the body with energy. Before the carbohydrates enter the blood, the body breaks down the ingested carbohydrates into glucose molecules.

The glucose molecules are then absorbed by the cells and used to produce adenosine triphosphate (ATP). Adenosine triphosphate serves as an energy supplier for numerous metabolic processes.

Most body cells can produce ATP not only from carbohydrates, but also from fats and, in exceptional cases, from amino acids.

However, the energy from carbohydrates is available to the body faster than from fats. For the production of ATP from fatty acids, the body needs sufficient oxygen.

From carbohydrates or glucose, the body can also produce ATP without oxygen. This is especially important for great effort, as oxygen is usually scarce. The body therefore uses fatty acids only at low to medium intensity and with prolonged activity.

If the body has more glucose available than it needs at the moment, it can store it in the liver or muscles. The storage form of glucose is called glycogen. About 100 grams of glycogen can be stored in the liver.

The body uses the glycogen stored in the liver either to generate energy or to keep blood sugar levels constant between meals.

The glycogen stores are not the only buffers that the body has to ensure the glucose supply of the body. If the body does not have enough glucose, it can convert amino acids into glucose and use them for energy supply. However, the breakdown of amino acids into glucose means that the body breaks down muscle mass.

This should be prevented as muscles are existential for any form of movement. The loss of muscle mass is also associated in scientific studies with an increased risk of disease.

Consuming at least some carbohydrates can prevent this state of glucose undersupply and prevent the breakdown of muscle mass as well as provide the brain with sufficient glucose.

Further possibilities for supplying the muscles with sufficient energy are presented in the following article.

The glycogen storage capacity of the muscle cells is about 500 grams. The glycogen, which is stored in the muscles, can only be used by the muscle cells themselves and is used for strenuous loads (2).

When all glycogen stores are filled, the body converts excess carbohydrates into triglycerides and stores them in the form of fat.

For example, oatmeal

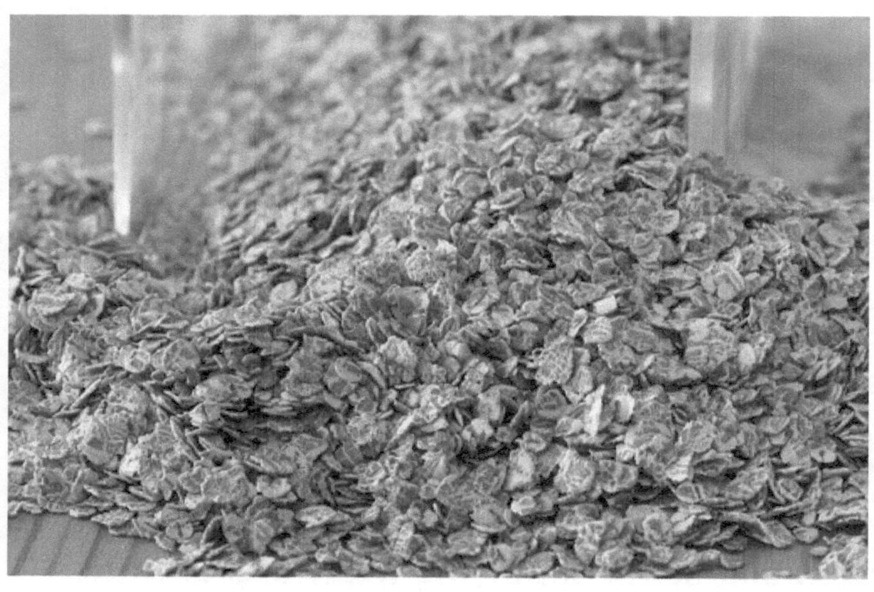

There are carbohydrates, the so-called fiber, which are not converted into glucose like starch or sugar, but pass through the intestines undigested. There is soluble and insoluble fiber.

Soluble fibre is contained, for example, in oatmeal, legumes, fruits or vegetables. They absorb water on the way through the intestine and form a gel-like substance.

Thus, the soluble fibers increase the stool volume and make the chair softer.

Insoluble fiberalsoes also increase the stool volume and also speed up the digestive process. They are contained in whole grains and in the shells of seeds, vegetables and fruits.

Scientific studies show that eating insoluble fiber can protect against some intestinal diseases.

For example, a study of 40,000 men found that regular consumption of insoluble fiber reduces the risk of developing diverticulosis by 37 percent.

Diverticulosis is an intestinal disease in which spouts form on the intestinal wall, which can become inflamed.

It can be noted that fiber promotes healthy digestion and gut health.

Do we need carbohydrates to live?

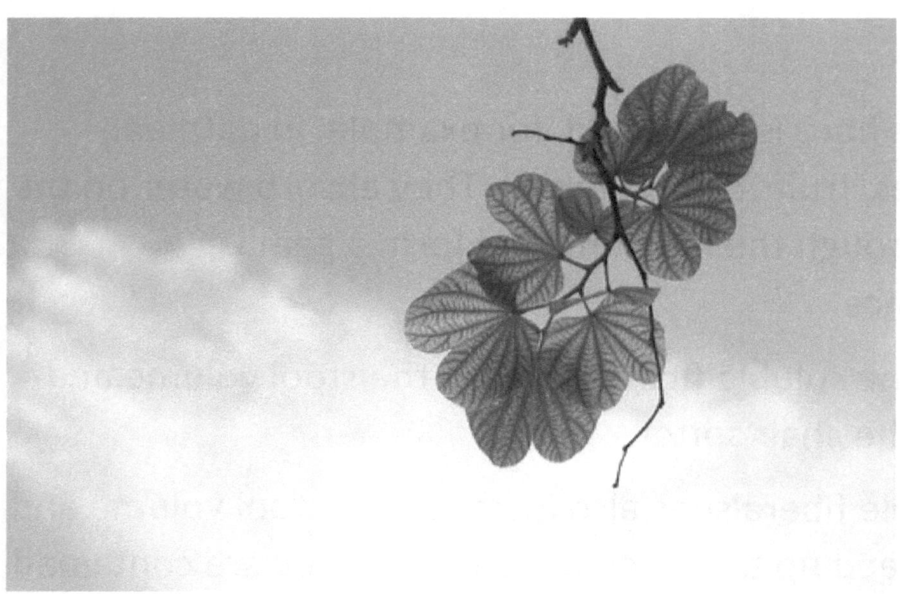

The provision of energy and the maintenance of muscles are among the most important functions of carbohydrates. Carbohydrates are not existential for the body, but can be replaced by other nutrients.

Virtually any body cell is able to produce ATP not only from carbohydrates, but also from fat. The largest energy storage in the human body is not the glycogen storage, but the adipose tissue.

Normally, the brain uses glucose as an energy supplier. In long periods of hunger or in an extremely low-carb diet, the brain also resorts to so-called ketone bodies.

Ketone bodies are formed during the splitting of fatty acids.

The body forms ketone bodies when it has no carbohydrates available for energy production. However, not all brain cells can use ketone bodies for energy production.

About a third of brain cells require glucose to generate energy. However, the body does not necessarily need carbohydrates for the required amount of glucose, as it can also make them from proteins

Before we come to the different sugar types and their respective labels or properties, it is now only necessary to clarify what the term "glycemic index" (GI) is all about:

The GI is a measure of the blood sugar-increasing effect of carbohydrate-rich foods.

Caution: It always refers to 50g carbohydrates/food, which is why it has misleading information on some foods.

Take, for example, the watermelon:

At 76, the GI is in a relatively high range

You see the GI can cause confusion from time to time. However, it should be taken seriously for the individual types of sugar, as sugars are pure carbohydrates.

Let's take a look at the concept of the "glycemic load" (GL).

The glycemic load is the extended form of the GI. Experts prefer the GL to the GI, as the glycemic load takes into account the amount of carbohydrates contained in the food.

Short-chain carbohydrates

Short-chain carbohydrates are, for example, glucose, fructose and galactose, where glucose from glucose is the most important energy source.

The simple sugar:

Glucose or dextrose

-easily water soluble

-mean sweetness of 69

-very easily digestible

-rest in the blood GI= approx. 120

Used for:

-Athlete's Nutrition

-Regulation of blood sugar levels

-Glucose syrup in sweets

-is an energy supplier for the brain

Is included in:

-Finished products

-Fruit

-cane and beet sugar

-Sweets

-Honey

Fruit sugar or fructose

-absorbed by the liver

-easily water soluble

-very high sweetness (approx. 120)

-goes relatively slowly into the blood

-GI corresponds to approx. 20

Used for:

-Diabetics, as it is digested insulin-independently*

- Additive of many finished products "glucose-fructose syrup"

Insulin is a hormone that transports nutrients from the blood into our cells and affects the feeling of hunger)

Is included in:

s.o. glucose

Fructose in industry ☹:

Markings:

Corn syrup

Glucose fructose syrup

Fruit sweetness

Fructose

<u>Disadvantages in the case of high intake</u>

Overweight

Fatty liver

Blood pressure

Insulin resistance

<u>Mucus sugar (galactose)</u>

-water soluble

-moderate sweetness (approx.63)

It is important for healthy development in infants

Occurrences it does in:

-Milk and cheese, as a component of lactose

-rarely occurs in free form

-is part of the mucous membranes

<u>The double sugar (disaccharides)</u>

Cane and beet sugar

(sucrose=our household sugar)

-water soluble

-Consists of one glucose molecule and one fructose molecule

-Sweetness is about 100

-must be split before absorption

-flows into the blood (GI=approx. 70)

Use:

-neutral-tasting sweetener

-for baking, sweetening, preserving

to happen:

-Addition in almost every highly processed food, in most in ready meals, confectionery

-natural occurrence: in dates, peaches, honey

Invert sugar = split sucrose:

-Mixture of equivalent glucose and fructose

-slightly less sweetness (approx. 93)

Used for cheap bakery production

Replacement for honey = "artificial honey"

Occurs in baked goods, honey, invert sugar cream, finished products, sweets

Lactose, lactose

-Consists of one molecule of glucose and galactose

-water soluble

-low sweetness (approx.39)

-flows leisurely into the blood

-GI is about 40

-promotes digestion

-requires the enzyme lactase for absorption

Used:

-to stimulate digestion in infants

-Diet food (milk powder), causes positive intestinal flora

Occurs in e.g. quark, yoghurt, cream cheese, milk

Malt sugar, maltose

-consists of two glucose molecules

-water soluble

-weak sweetness of approx. 46

-goes quickly into the blood, GI = approx. 100

Used as a basis for beer production

Occurs in e.g. beer, cereal malt, malt coffee, coating at cornflakes

<u>The multiple sugars (=oligosaccharides)</u>

These include:

-Raffinosis (Gal, Glu, Woman)

-Stachyose (Gal, Glu, Woman)

-Oligofructose (woman)

They are used in sports nutrition and dietary foods.

Come before in:

-Breast milk - longer saturation

-Legumes (raffinosis)

-Artichokes (Stachyose)

-Garlic (oligofructose)

<u>Multiple sugar (=polysaccharides)</u>

These include:

Dextrin

-consist of 10- several 1000 monosaccharide residues

-are degradation products of starch

-consist only of glucose molecules

-well water soluble

-taste weak sweet

-easier to digest as strength

-do not provide energy as fast as glucose

-when heated at temperatures of approx. 150°C

Such as. When baking bread (bread crust) - give colour and taste

use in energy bars, dietary foods such as maltodextrin for a build-up diet

<u>Are included in:</u>

-Pastry crusts

-Toast

-Zwieback

Cellulose

-is one of the insoluble fibres

-consists of more than 10,000 glucose residues

-is water insoluble

-no sweet taste

-fibrous, solid substance

-low swelling capacity

-stimulates digestion

Cellulose is the substance of plant cells,

therefore, it is found in cereals, fruit and vegetables.

The same applies to

Hemicellulose

-located between the fibrils of the cellulose

-is difficult to insoluble in water

-swells more than cellulose but lower than pectins

-is digestive

<u>Pectins</u>

-include soluble fibres

-consists of about 35 glucose residues

-dissolve gel-like in hot water - gels can bind

-bind cholesterol and excrete it

-very good swelling ability

-insoluble in cold water

-supply no energy

-acts on e.g. jam as gelling agent

Pectins are components of plant cell walls

-used as thickeners in the LM industry

-occur in core fruit, e.g. apples, quinces

-in berry fruit e.g. raspberries

-part of gelling sugar

<u>Strength</u>

It consists of:

Amylose (200-1000 glucose molecules) = spiral arrangement of molecules

Amylopectin (600-6000 glucose molecules) = strongly branched structure of molecules

<u>Strength is located in:</u>

-Baked goods, Teigen

-Pudding, or pudding powder

-Sweets

-Potatoes

-Cereals

The GI depends on the food from which the starch is obtained

<u>Carbohydrate is not equal to carbohydrate</u>

There are carbohydrates that are better for the balance of our body than others.

The more complex a carbohydrate is, the longer it takes our body to break it down into its constituents and bring the sugar molecules into the bloodstream. The sweeter a product tastes, the higher the proportion of simple carbohydrates and the faster the sugar molecules that are contained go into the blood. For example, if we eat a doughnut or just a spoonful of household sugar, the blood sugar level rises rapidly.

In response, the pancreas releases insulin, and blood sugar levels quickly drop again. The body signals "memory empty", so we are hungry again quickly.

If, on the other hand, we eat a piece of wholemeal bread or a bowl of natural rice, the complex carbohydrates contained in it must first be disassembled and are only gradually available to the body. The blood sugar curve is flatter, and we stay full longer.

What is the low-carb diet?

As the name suggests, the low-carb diet promises to reduce weight by taking "carbs" (the English word Carbohydrates).

A feature of the diet is therefore to compose all meals with as much saturating protein as possible and to avoid carbohydrates especially in the evening.

This eliminates products such as traditional pasta, potatoes and bread and is replaced by fish, meat, cheese and other dairy products, as well as vegetables and nuts.

Just through low-carbohydrate foods. And those who now think they have to remove their beloved noodles from the menu forever have been far from it, because: Low carb is not the same as "no carb".

The low-carb diet is probably so successful because it is not designed in the short term. On the contrary, the low-carb diet is by no means a crash diet, but a healthy and lasting diet change.

You can find out exactly how the diet works, which foods you should absolutely avoid and what alternatives our supermarkets have in store.

The principle is to consume low carbohydrates

So those who reduce cereal products and potatoes and replace them with low-carbohydrate foods will soon be able to look forward to customer succession.

How does low-carb diet work?

As mentioned above, it is not advisable to turn a low-carb diet into a no-carb diet. However, a distinction should be made between complex and simple carbohydrates:

Products with complex carbohydrates contain a lot of fiber, keep full for a long time and are an important digestive promoter. These include whole grains, legumes and whole grains. Depending on how hurried you want to lose weight, a low-carb diet allows 20-100 grams of complex carbohydrates per day.

However, you should avoid simple carbohydrates such as sugar, white bread, soft drinks, rolls, pizza and classic pasta.

These carbohydrates are quickly broken down by the body and transported by the body into the cells with the help of more produced insulin. Unfortunately, insulin inhibits fat burning and ensures that fat is stored in the abdominal area with preference.

In addition, the rapid increase in insulin levels causes our blood sugar to drop rapidly, which is noticeable in our case in the form of craving attacks.

These foods are prohibited at low-carb!

We have compiled for you which foods specifically belong to the "tabu" products of a low-carb diet in a small overview:

Pasta made from wheat flour: The exception, as mentioned above, are products made from whole grains or oatmeal, which are allowed in small quantities.

Pasta and Co.: Overall, a high consumption of carbohydrate-containing foods such as rice, potatoes, pasta and bread must be avoided.

Carbohydrate-containing fruit: Fruit is not the same as fruit. There are varieties that have a very high carbohydrate content and should be better avoided in a low-carb diet. These include, for example: bananas, grapes and raisins.

Cereals and breakfast cereals: Classic cereals from the supermarket often have a very high carbohydrate content due to a lot of sugar. That's why these products haven't lost anything in a low-carb diet.

Sugar: Since sugar is 100 percent carbohydrates, sugar should no longer be on the menu. This also includes soft drinks, fruit juices, sweets and baked goods of all kinds.

You can eat these foods without any worries

There are so many foods on the "allowed" list of the low-carb diet that we can't list them in detail. For a better overview, the table below

Vegetables and mushrooms

You don't have to be shy here. Vegetables have hardly any calories, but provide a lot of fiber and digestion is encouraged. To compensate for the missing carbohydrates, you should fill your plate generously, preferably with water-rich vegetables. This fills you quickly and sustainably, and only slowly raises blood sugar levels.

In addition, vegetables, phytochemicals that have a positive effect on heart health.

Vegetables
Carbohydrates in grams per 100 grams
Mushrooms
0,8
Fresh leaf spinach
0,6
Sauerkraut
0,8

Chinese cabbage
0,8
Lettuce
1,0
Cucumber
2,0
Zucchini
2,0

Meat and fish

These foods provide you with the protein you need. On the one hand, protein provides a pleasant feeling of satiety, on the other hand, protein also helps your body to build muscle and boosts metabolism. Do not pay too much attention to the fat content, because the omega-3 fatty acids in fish and meat also protect the heart and vessels.

If possible, you should pay attention to animals and their health to love, if possible, products from animal welfare. Most meats and fish contain very little to no carbohydrates.

Low sugar fruit

Perfect for a low-carb diet are fruit varieties that have only a low carbohydrate content. Therefore, prefer to use berry fruit, kiwis, watermelon, avocados, apples, pears and citrus fruits.

Fruit
Carbohydrates in grams per 100 grams
Avocado
2,0
Lemon
3,0
Blackberries/Rasberries/Cranberries
5,0
Watermelon
6,0
Kiwi
8,0
Apple
11,0
Pear
11,0

Dairy products

Here, too, the high protein content has the positive saturating effect. Dairy products also score with bone-strengthening calcium, vitamin D, zinc, iodine and vitamin A.

However, when it came to processed products, you should always have a look at the ingredients contained therein. Sugar is mainly added to fruit yoghurts.

Dairy products
Carbohydrates in grams per 100 grams
Harz cheese
0
granular cream cheese
1,1
Cottage cheese
3,3
Greek yoghurt 10%
4,3
Yoghurt 0.1%
5,8
Tofu and Co.

The protein products listed below are particularly suitable for the vegetarian low-carb eaters. It should be noted that these products are very heavily processed and are taken as meat substitutes:

Tofu
Carbohydrates in grams per 100 grams
Smoked tofu
1,0
Tofu
2,0

Eggs are a real miracle cure! They are super versatile, a pleasure at any time of the day and provide you with protein as well as fat-soluble vitamins such as A, D and E.

So, an absolute must for the low-carb diet. You can find out below why you don't usually have to be afraid of the high level of cholesterol when eating eggs.

Carbohydrates in grams per 100 grams
Yolk
0
Egg - Full egg
1,0

<table>
<tr><td>Protein/egg white</td></tr>
<tr><td>1,0</td></tr>
</table>

Fats and oils

Although meat and therefore animal fats play an overriding role in the low-carb diet, you should also resort to vegetable fats during the diet. For example, plant-based oils such as olive, rapeseed, walnut and coconut oil. They ensure a smooth metabolism and good fat burning.

Fats and oils, the special thing about it is:

These foods do not contain carbohydrates

Butter

Coconut

Pumpkin seed oil

Linseed oil

Rapeseed oil

Olive oil

Nuts

For snacking and snacking and also for cooking – almonds, Brazil nuts, macadamia nuts and walnuts as well as pine nuts and flaxseeds are rich in antioxidant vitamin E and complement the low-carb diet excellently.

Nuts and seeds may have a percentage of carbohydrates. This carbohydrate content is usually very low:

Low carbohydrate content for nuts, seeds and seeds

Pumpkin seeds

Flaxseed

Brazil nuts

Chia seeds

Macadamia

Almonds

Pecans

Walnuts

Due to the high fat content and high energy density, please nevertheless consider a controlled consumption, and appropriate amounts of these foods

Benefits of the Low-Carb Diet

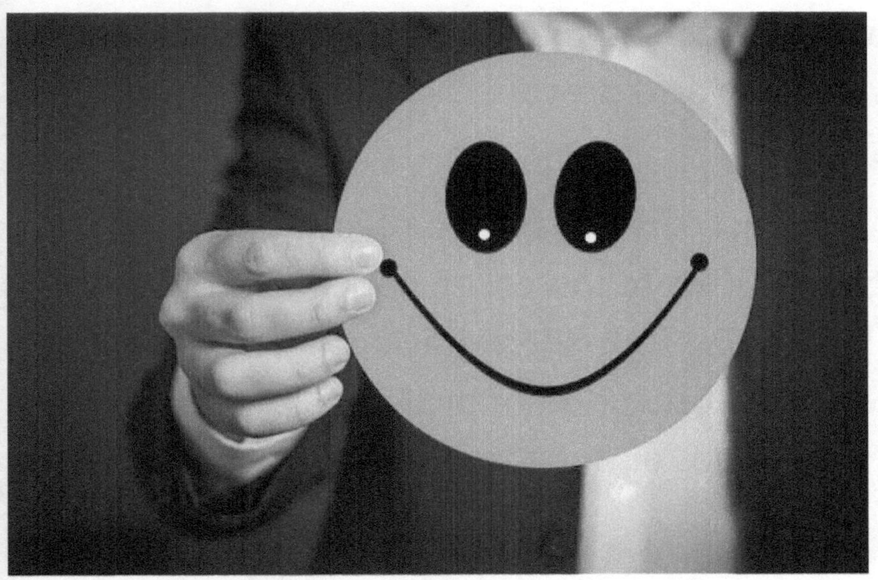

A clear advantage of the low-carb diet lies in its simplicity:

No calories need to be counted and the list of foods that should be avoided is quickly understandable. You will also deal with the topic of nutrition and get a feeling for the main nutrient's fat, protein and carbohydrates – so overall a better awareness of food and the needs of your body.

Our body, if you look at its main nutrients, actually still lives in the Stone Age. Especially the many sugars of today, makes our health and our body difficult. The low-carb diet helps you maintain healthy blood sugar levels, which can also prevent diseases such as diabetes.

Last but not least, the advantage of low-carb nutrition may be that it leads to increased concentration and positive well-being (provided they eat a balanced diet). In addition, the absorption of proteins, fats and fiber, through vegetables and meat, prevents craving attacks.

Disadvantages in low-carb diet, usually only with one-sided diet

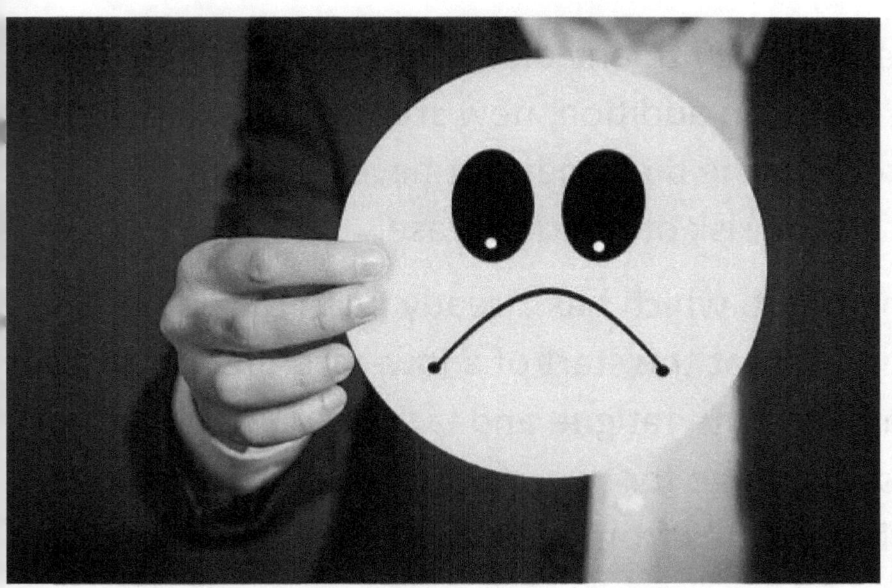

Many scientists criticize the strict renunciation of carbohydrates, as this can lead to malnutrition and malnutrition as well as irritation of the psyche. However, this thesis presupposes that those people only eat red meat, eggs and unnatural protein shakes during the low-carb diet. This is usually too one-sided.

A low-carb diet should always be balanced. With the help of enough vegetables and additionally small portions of complex carbohydrates, deficiency symptoms are unlikely.

Furthermore, the risk of heart disease is associated with low-carb diet. The low-carb diet is also high in cholesterol and fat, which many people see as a disadvantage of the diet. Again, everything applies in moderation!

Balance is the key to any diet and also applies to the low-carb diet. In addition, new studies have shown that cholesterol in the diet does not have a significant impact on the risk of heart disease.

Also, the point, which has already been raised here many times, that the start of a low-carb diet often goes hand in hand with fatigue and lack of drive should not be a disadvantage for you. You don't have to remove the carbohydrates from your diet overnight.

With a slow weaning over several days or weeks, i.e. a slow reduction of carbs, such side effects can be avoided.

Conclusion to a healthy and balanced lifestyle

The most important point, which is and remains a healthy diet, i.e. to eat in a varied way and to focus more on plant-based foods.

With a balanced and varied diet, the risk of deficiency symptoms decreases considerably.

Immediately after that, the point is **to enjoy** the food and take your time with the **food.** What I eat should **also taste and** make me full.

Scientists have found that a slow chewing and generally delayed eating process causes faster saturation.

In the end, this means that we are more likely to eat smaller people and thus consume fewer calories.

A sufficient supply of liquid is also very important. Water, unsweetened teas, coffee or other calorie-free drinks are suitable. In fact, I do not think that fruit juices are recommended either. Instead, consuming an entire fruit simply provides more health-relevant nutrients, and also takes longer than a glass of juice.

Drinking amounts of up to 2.5l per day are recommended. Athletes and pregnant people, can and should drink up to 500ml more.

Since the revelation of the cholesterol myth or the deferral of the bad reputation of the fat-like substance cholesterol, experts have changed the minds regarding the consumption of the main nutrient fat.

Cholesterol was suspected of being consumed too frequently and in excessive amounts, increasing the risk of cardiovascular disease and atherosclerosis.

Cholesterol-dangerous?

It is now known that the organism can control cholesterol levels. The body itself produces amounts of cholesterol every day. If cholesterol is now fed through the diet, the body regulates this by lowering the body's own production. The morning breakfast egg is back in the game!

It is important to note, however, that people who have elevated cholesterol levels due to illness-related circumstances should exercise caution. It is best to discuss with a doctor about future cholesterol consumption.

Fat should and must be back on the menu.

In particular, vegetable fats should be preferred, which have a favorable fatty acid pattern mentioned above.

It is also important to pay attention to what I use for which fat. Some oils cannot be heated too high, and therefore form substances that are harmful to health at elevated temperatures.

A still current problem is the consumption of sugar in society. Even if you look at the balance sheets of sugar consumption over the past few years, it is not possible to draw any conclusions about a permanent and significant decline. Low sugar consumption should be taken into account because it is in almost all foods, but it provides nothing but energy, which ultimately leads us to increased weight levels or increased fat mass due to insufficient activity.

Meat and fish consumption in moderation

Consumption of meat and fish and their products should still be within a moderate framework.

Consumption of mainly fatty fish favours the daily fatty acid pattern due to the essential fatty acids it contains. In addition, meat and fish often provide a high concentration of proteins.

When meat is eaten, lean or low-fat varieties should be preferred. Care should be taken with red meat, it usually contains a lot of saturated fat, as well as a high proportion of purines and cholesterol, whereby cholesterol poses a danger only to certain individuals as mentioned above.

However, animal foods, such as milk and dairy products, should be consumed daily due to the high calcium content. Calcium is 99% stored in our bones and is only present in very low concentrations in the free metabolism. The calcium in bones, is built up until the thirtieth year of life, or stored. After this period, the body begins to gradually break down these calcium stores. That sounds worse at first.

Up to 1000mg of calcium should be absorbed daily until the age of 30 to store sufficient supplies. In athletes, pregnant women and the elderly, this need can increase slightly.

Eat vegetables and fruit more often

Larger quantities of vegetables and, if necessary, fruit are recommended. Due to the vitamins, nutrients and minerals as well as fiber, these foods strengthen our health, and help with weight loss, through a faster saturation.

Vegetables should occur several times in meals that are consumed during the day. In the case of fruit, the often-high sugar content must be taken into account. Especially the fructose in apples, for example, can cause problems in some people.

According to current recommendations, the whole grain variant should always be chosen for cereal products. This would saturate longer and bring with it significantly higher nutrient concentrations than white flour products.

In addition, whole grain products reduce the risk of type 2 diabetes mellitus, colorectal cancer, cardiovascular disease and fat metabolism disorders

The advice to consume plenty of carbohydrates in the form of cereal products and potatoes should no longer be taken into account. Experts had long criticized that such a diet makes losing weight more difficult and favors diabetes.

Mistakes made again and again in a diet

Next, we'll look at the factors that make your goal difficult and stubbornly anchor you

People rely only on the scales

Those who weigh themselves daily can quickly be disappointed. The number does not change fast enough, although all diet rules are adhered to. But what many forget:

Weight is influenced by several different factors, including fluid balance or how much food is still in the digestive tract.

The weight can vary by about 1.4 kilograms per day. In women, other factors such as a change in hormone levels, which can lead to increased water retention and thus reflect as more on the scale, play a role.

As already mentioned, the number on the scale also depends on whether muscles are built up. Because fat is burned during muscle growth, but this is not necessarily visible on the scale. This can be frustrating despite the loss of weight.

If you want to lose weight without frustration, don't just use a scale to capture your weight loss process. Take your measurements every now and then, especially the hip circumference is important here. Before-and-after photos can also help to see the customer's order more clearly.

Too hasty and impatient

Another problem with losing weight is unrealistic expectations. This relates both to the objective and to the time it is to be achieved.

Every body is different. This means that not everyone can reach a certain body shape. Especially on the Internet, beauty ideals are haunting, which are completely unrealistic and can be achieved with no diet or sports program.

Losing weight takes time: Losing weight does not go from today to morning. You don't get the same fat within twenty-four hours.

Expecting to reach the desired weight and the dream body within a very short time is completely unrealistic. According to one study, those with the highest expectations are most likely to cancel a diet or a diet program.

Setting a goal is important for weight loss success and can usually motivate. However, set realistic goals that can be logical and don't plunge into unhealthy crash diets without a plan. This not only preserves motivation in the long term, but also does not harm your psyche.

No knowledge of ingredients

If you want to lose weight, you have to be aware of what you are eating. It is advantageous to take a close look at the packaging of food and read the list of ingredients and the nutritional information. If necessary, you can then also deal with this information a little more and, for example, do research on the Internet. Otherwise, it can happen quickly that you eat unwanted kilocalories or rather unhealthy ingredients for the body.

This can be particularly disastrous for products that are supposedly healthy or claim this on the packaging. In this way, the buyer is tricked into believing that there is a false security. Caution should also be exercised with diet and light products, as many low-fat yoghurts often hide appetizing sweeteners and many additives.

No sport

If you lose weight, you don't just kill fat. Muscle mass is also used by the organism to gain energy due to lack of energy. The proportion of muscle degraded depends on various factors. For example, if you don't do sports, you will lose more muscle mass and, as a result, have a lower basic turnover.

On the other hand, those who exercise will lose less muscle mass. With increased fat-free muscle mass, it is easier to lose weight and keep the weight constant over a long period of time.

But there is also too much of sport. This in turn is stressful for the body. Excessive exposure to exercise can exhaust the adrenal glands and produce fewer adrenal hormones that regulate stress levels and thus reduce cortisol.

Many people also make the mistake of losing weight to overestimate the kilocalorie consumption during a sports session. Sport increases the basic turnover, but not as much as you might think. When jogging, for example, you consume about 350 kilocalories in half an hour.

A study by the University of Ottawa showed that people who burned about 200 to 300 kilocalories during a sports session estimated their consumption at more than 800 kilocalories. So, they ate more and consumed more kilocalories – so they didn't reach the calorie deficit they actually wanted.

It is also important to mention that this is a pure endurance training, which is not necessarily productive for losing weight.

Often only endurance sports are associated with weight loss – those who struggle on the treadmill also burn a lot of fat. In fact, strength training is also one of the most important ways to lose weight. Because the lean muscle mass is decisive for a loss of weight.

Even a physically stressful workout, so a strength training, can significantly reduce the path to the dream body.

Studies have even shown that strength training is one of the most effective ways to build muscle and optimize metabolism. In addition, it is beneficial for the entire body composition and helps to burn abdominal fat. The best results are achieved when endurance and strength training are combined.

Pay attention to a mixture of endurance and strength training and watch out for signals from your body.

More muscle mass, burns more calories

Losing weight is about being under-calorie for a longer period of time. In the case of a calorie deficit, however, it should be noted that the basic turnover, i.e. the energy that the body needs to maintain its functions and provide the internal organs with nutrients, should always be covered. However, in order to increase the consumption of energy, exercise helps, i.e. an intensive training. With increasing muscles, the basic consumption and energy consumption in training increase. A person with a high muscle content thus consumes significantly more kilocalories at rest and in exercise than a person with rather untrained less muscles. In theory, this leads to a more effective decline. Again, it should be noted that losing weight does not always mean weight loss, as a higher muscle density weighs more than the same volume of fat.

The greatest successes in losing weight are achieved through a combination of endurance and strength training. Strength training is even one of the most effective methods of losing weight.

Too high calorie deficit, too little energy

As already mentioned, a calorie deficit is necessary to reduce. Until now, a deficit of 3500 kilocalories per week can result in a weight loss of about half a kilo per week. A recent study by Montclair State University found that this statement is not to be generalized, but varies from person to person.

To burn one kilo of fat, 7000 kilocalories must be burned. Although fat per gram has an energy density of 9kcal, some of the energy is lost during the metabolic process.

It is important to mention that with an extreme calorie deficit, the metabolism is reduced or the metabolic rate is reduced, so the body is practically in saving mode, and therefore the basic turnover is also reduced.

Too many calories

Many underestimates their daily calorie intake. In one study, ten obese people, i.e. more than average overweight people, reported having consumed 1,000 kilocalories a day during the test phase. Subsequent investigations, however, revealed that they actually consumed about twice the number of kilocalories.

Another typical mistake in losing weight is to consider healthy foods per se to be "good". Healthy foods that are very high in calories, such as nuts or cheese, can also make you fat.

Get off to a good weight: The portion size is crucial. Find out how much your personal daily turnover is, and follow it. A nutrition diary can be helpful to keep track

This always applies:

Only a calorie deficit can lose weight, but this should not be too large, as this is unhealthy. A nutrition diary can help to record the daily calorie intake.

Fiber is neglected

An undersupply of fibre is becoming more and more common.

Fiber requires a lot of chewing, and is in hand with increased saliva production. As a result, chewing in fiber-containing foods is used for longer. In addition, a faster saturation occurs with a consumption of fiber.

Foods with a high fiber content are slow to raise blood sugar levels – this prevents craving attacks. Water-soluble fiber, such as pectins, form a gel with water. In addition, they have a positive effect on blood sugar levels.

In addition, fiber helps the body absorb and store fewer amounts of fat because it slows down some certain fat-splitting enzymes at work.

Integrating high-fiber foods such as cereals, legumes, vegetables and fruits into your diet helps you get a good step closer to the goal.

In summary, fiber can cause a long feeling of satiety and can help the body absorb and store less fat.

During a diet you should eat many proteins. These can support weight loss by providing a faster satiety feeling, thus largely curbing appetite, reducing calorie intake and stimulating metabolism. In addition, less muscle mass is obviously broken down if the body receives enough proteins through the diet.

An increased use of plant proteins in the diet is very important, as has been mentioned several times. We note that proteins are generally very important during weight loss. Much less muscle mass is broken down and these proteins have an appetizing effect, saturating and stimulate metabolism and fat burning.

Eat too often

There are also various views on how many meals should be eaten a day. Whether many small or three large main meals – the right eating behavior should prevent a strong feeling of hunger. However, if you adhere too strictly to these rules, you may absorb more kilocalories than you actually need, as you no longer trust your own feelings.

In principle, it is recommended to eat intuitively. It is really important to look at yourself individually. So, listen to your gut feeling when eating and pay attention to the natural feeling of satiety. So, you shouldn't feel obliged to have breakfast, or to keep a certain amount of meals, even if someone recommends that.

A common mistake in losing weight is to restrict yourself too much and to completely remove food from your own diet. A renunciation of whole food groups can also have a negative effect on the psyche. In any case, care should be taken to approve something rather "unhealthy", such as a small portion of sweets, in order to strengthen motivation and stamina. For example, when you reach a specific sub-goal, imagine embedsing a small "sin." Here, of course, it is important to take this system to a small and small extent.

Calories in liquid form

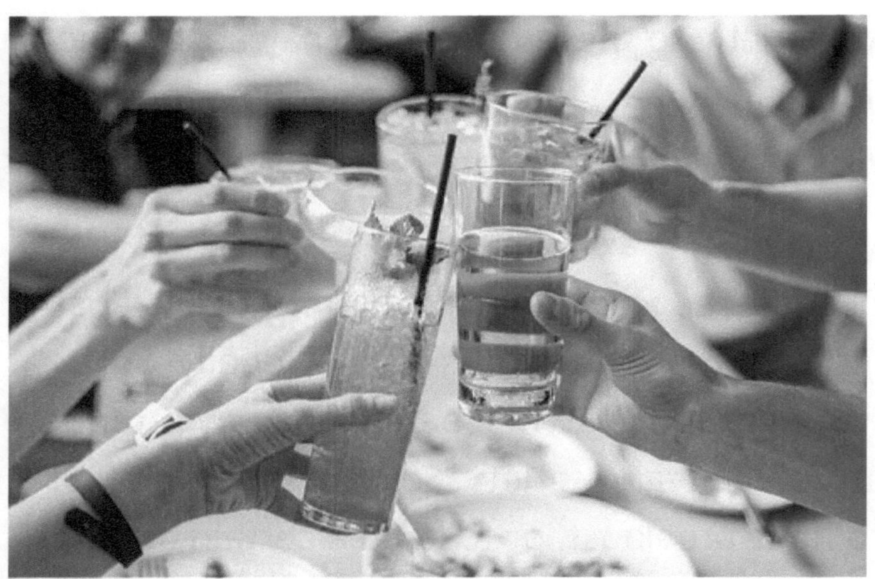

Liquid calories, our body easily utilises. You only get satisfied if you drink so much that your stomach is filled. Liquid calories are rapidly transferred to the metabolism, and are therefore quickly utilized by the organism. So, as a conclusion, saturated drinks are not as much as solid food. You can absorb kilocalories, but you don't feel the same feeling of satiety as after eating a solid snack. As a result, more kilocalories are absorbed so often because the sugary drink is not compensated by giving up other foods.

Although many people who want to lose weight already do without sugary soft drinks and calorie-containing otherwise sweetened drinks and thus save many kilocalories. However, it is often forgotten and neglected that the supposedly healthy fruit juice also contains a lot of natural sugar – also natural pressed commercial goods with a fruit content of 100%.

Beverages that carry vitamins and minerals can have the same weight effects as drinks with industrial sugar.

The consumption of alcohol must also be observed.

At 7kcal/g, alcohol contains almost as many calories as fat. In addition, the consumption of alcohol leads to a decrease in the metabolic rate, as the body is busy reducing the "poison". With frequent alcohol consumption, the body's basic turnover decreases again.

Eating highly processed foods

Another mistake in losing weight is to eat many rather industrially processed foods.

Several studies have already shown that these foods can often lead to overweight or obesity and various other health problems such as headaches, gastrointestinal discomfort or diabetes. Therefore, it is recommended to use natural foods that are produced without additives and therefore cannot affect the natural feeling of satiety.

As a conclusion, we draw from this that processed foods often lead to obesity and health problems, as they contain many unknown additives that are not really relevant to health.

Instead, fresh, full-fledged food should be preferred, preferably unprocessed food.

At the end of this book, a few sportsmen and low carb recipes that especially help women lose weight:

Low-Carb-Kitchen

Breakfast:

Low-carb pancakes:

Ingredients for 4-5 pancakes:

2	Egg (er)
125 g	Hazelnuts, ground
5 ml	Sweetener, liquid
2 TB	Flour or protein powder
1 tsp, yesterday.	Cinnamon powder
n. B.	Whole milk, 3.5% fat
1 pinch(s)	Salt
	Oil, for frying
Possibly.	Cinnamon powder, for sprinkling

Preparation:

Working time approx. 20 min. cooking time approx. 10 min. Total time approx. 30 min.

Put the eggs, hazelnuts, sweetener, flour, cinnamon, milk and salt in a mixing bowl and mix well with an electric hand stirrer.

The amount of milk should be chosen in such a way that a thick but not too solid "porridge" is created.

Put a soup bowl full of dough in a hot, oil-greased pan and fry the pancakes golden brown from both sides, but make sure the temperature of the pan is not too high.

Low-carb muesli

Ingredients for 12 portions:

200 g	*Coconut rasp*
100 g	*Almonds, ground*
100 g	*Sunflower*
50 g	*Walnuts*
50 g	*Pumpkin seeds*
20 g	*Protein powder, chocolate flavor*
20 g	*Cocoa powder, 60% cocoa content*
4	*Protein*
	Sweetener, or stevia

Preparation:

Working time approx. 10 min. cooking time approx. 60 min. Total time approx. 70 min.

Put all the dry ingredients in a bowl and mix together. Mix the egg whites with sweetener or stevia and add to the bowl. Mix well together to create a homogeneous and uniformly moist mass. It should all be slightly crumbly.

Line a

baking tray with baking paper and spread the mixture evenly. For 60 min, slide into the oven preheated to 130 degrees. Every 15 min everything should be mixed well again, so that the drying takes place evenly. Since the mass is quite productive, spread the whole thing on two baking sheets.

Allow to cool well after baking and fill in a suitable box or container.

Die fertigen Pfannkuchen nach Belieben noch mit etwas

Zimt bestreuen.

Low-carb bread with sunflower seeds:

Ingredients for 1 bread:

50 g	Sunflower
50 g	Flaxseed, scraped
50 g	Wheat bran
50 g	Protein powder, neutral taste
2	Egg(er), size M
250 g	Skimmed quark
1 tsp, heaped	Baking powder
1 TT	Salt

Preparation:

Working time approx. 10 min. rest period approx. 10 min. Cooking/baking time approx. 40 min. Total time approx. 60 min.

Preheat the oven to 200°C.

Mix the dry ingredients, add the quark and eggs and knead a dough. Let the dough draw for 10 minutes. The flaxseeds then swell and the dough becomes a little firmer. Form a loaf of bread and bake for about 40 minutes.

I just use a baking paper on a rust.

If you like, you can cut the bread with a knife before baking, quietly a little deeper, about 1 cm, and sprinkle with sunflower seeds and, if necessary, press them a little. But that's only for the optics.

Other seeds/seeds or nuts can also be used for this recipe, provided that there are few carbohydrates.

Quark bread low carb:

Ingredients for 1 serving:

2 larges	Egg (er)
500 g	Skimmed quark
300 g	Almonds, ground
50 g	Chia seeds
5 g	Baking powder
1 TT	Psyllium
1 TT	Salt

Preparation:

Working time approx. 10 min. cooking time approx. 60 min. Total time approx. 70 min.

Mix all ingredients and bake at 180 degrees circulating air for about an hour.

If you don't mind a calorie increase here, you can add some nuts, such as walnuts and or hazelnuts, to the ingredients.

Coffee Cream Low Carb:

Ingredients:

2 TB	Soy milk (soy drink)
1 tbsp, yesterday.	Coffee powder, instant
20 g	Scattersweet with stevia
150 g	Soy quark (quark alternative), unsweetened
1 TT	Cinnamon powder
1/2 Cup	Cardamom powder
½ Cup	Carnation powder
1/2 spoon	Vanilla paste
5g	Cocoa powder, unsweetened
5g	Soy cream (soy cream cuisine)

Preparation:

Working time approx. 20 min. rest period approx. 120 min. Total time approx. 140 min.

Mix the soy milk, coffee powder and sprinklesweets together and heat on a medium level until the coffee powder is completely dissolved. Then pour into a large bowl and add the soy quark. Mix thoroughly until a homogeneous mass is formed. Add the cinnamon, vanilla paste, cardamom and clove powder and season to taste. Mix well again and leave in the fridge for at *least 2 hours. Garnish with unsweetened cocoa powder and soy cream.*

Tip: It is best to prepare the coffee cream the night before and enjoy it the next morning.

Stracciatella orange quark cream:

Ingredients for 1 serving:

250 g	*Skimmed quark*
1	*Orange(s)*
10 g	*Dark chocolate, grated*
1/2 TL	*Cinnamon*
10 g	*Coconut rasp*

| 10 g | Coconut |
| 1 shot | Mineral water with carbonic acid |

Preparation:

Working time approx. 10 min. Total time approx. 10 min.

Peel and dice the orange. Put the skimmed quark in a bowl with all the other ingredients and mix well. Finally, add the orange pieces.

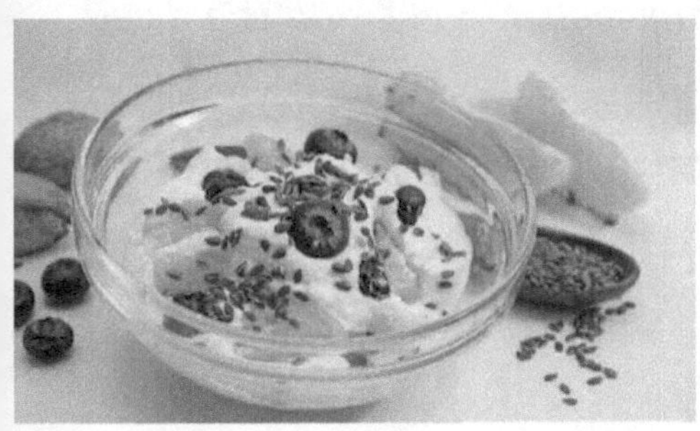

Nut apple quark cream:

Ingredients for 1 serving:

250 g	Skimmed quark
30g	Nuts of choice
1	Apple
1/2 TL	Cinnamon
10 g	Almond leaves

| 10 g | Peanuts |
| 1 shot | Mineral water with carbonic acid |

Preparation:

Working time approx. 10 min. Total time approx. 10 min.

Peel and dice the apple if necessary. Put the skimmed quark and all the remaining ingredients on the almond leaves in a bowl and mix well. Finally, add the diced apple.

Bananas or other fruits and nuts are also great for this

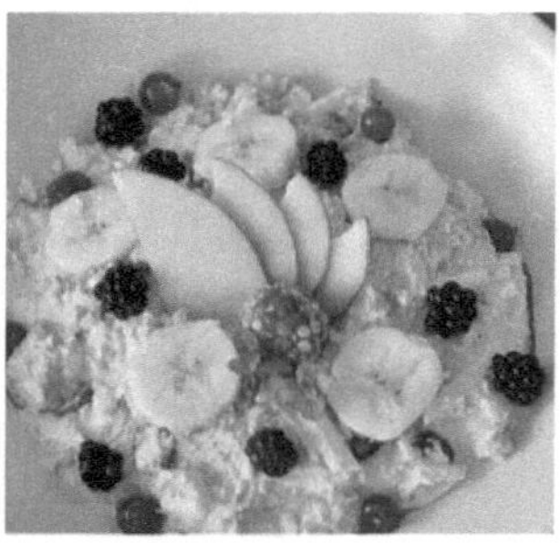

Pineapple chia pudding low carb:

Ingredients for 1 serving:

| 30 g | Chia seeds |
| 60 g | Coconut milk without added sugar |

80 g	Pineapple
10 g	Coconut
20 g	chopped nuts
120 ml	Water

Preparation:

Working time approx. 5 min. Total time approx. 5 min.

Puree the chia seeds in the blender. Add all the remaining ingredients and mix until everything is well mixed.

Either enjoy the pudding immediately or chill in the fridge, and eat a little later or the next morning.

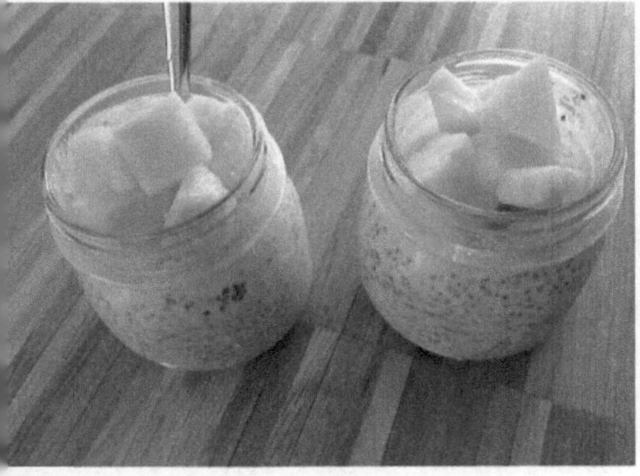

Fruity cottage cheese breakfast with nuts:

Ingredients for 1 serving:

200 g	Cream cheese, granular
50g	Blueberries or fruit to taste
30g	Nuts (nut mixture)
1 TB	Almonds, chopped
3 drops	Liquid sweetener
1 pinch(s)	Cinnamon powder
something	Nuts for garnish

Preparation:

Working time approx. 10 min. Total time approx. 10 min.

Put the granular cream cheese in a bowl. Add a handful of the nut mixture and mix.

Put a handful of fruit in a high container, with me it was blueberries and puree. Stir in a splash of liquid sweetener and add the granular cream cheese. Decorate with the nuts and chopped almonds and sprinkle with a pinch of cinnamon.

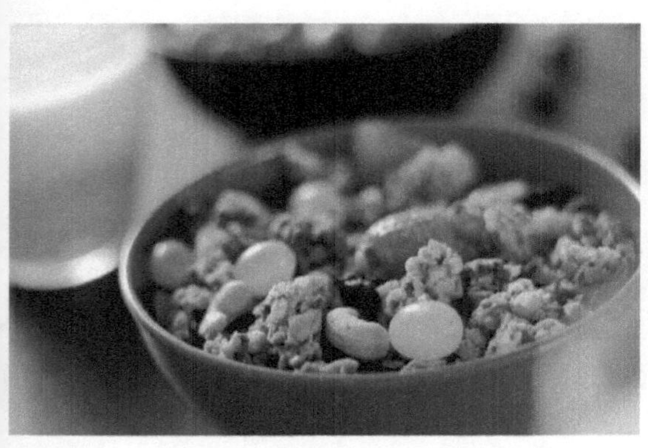

Low Carb Flame Cake

Ingredients for 1 flame cake:

250 g	*Cauliflower florets*
2 m.-sized	*Egg (er)*
200 g	*Cheese, grated*
1 cup	*Creme fra'che*
1 m.-large	*Onion(s)*
1 small	*Paprikaschote(s)*
	Salt and pepper

Preparation:

Working time approx. 10 min. cooking time approx. 40 min. Total time approx. 50 min.

For the bottom, finely rasp the raw cauliflower so that the consistency is reminiscent of small rice grains. Then add the eggs and 150 g of grated cheese and lightly salt. Mix the ingredients to create a slightly crumbly mass.

Cover a

sheet of baking paper and place the dough in a round shape using a spring-frying edge. This can be done very easily with your hands. Make sure that there are no holes in the bottom of the dough. Bake the dough prepared in the oven (circulating air: 180 °C, upper/under heat: 160 °C) for 25 minutes.

In the meantime, for the topping, mix the cream with the remaining cheese, salt and pepper, cut the onion into thin rings and the peppers into fine strips.

Now sprinkle the pre-baked soil with the cream-fra'che mixture, cover with onions and peppers and bake in the oven for another 15 minutes.

Can be documented with all sorts of things:

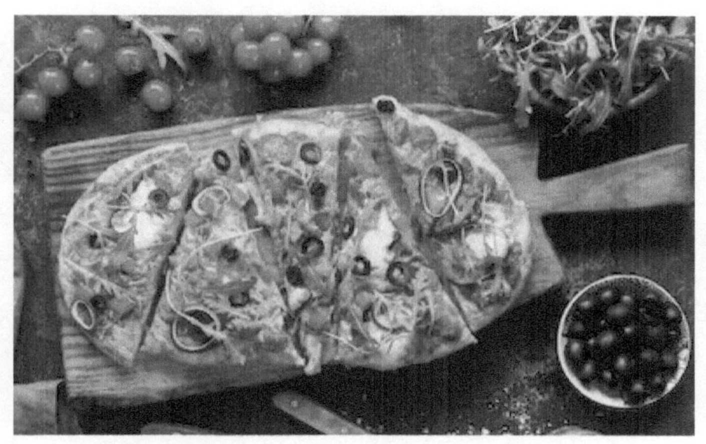

Low-carb cheese roll

Ingredients for 1 serving:

125 g	*Skimmed quark*
1/4 Pck.	*grated cheese approx. 50 g*
2	*Egg (er)*

For the sauce:

1 TT	*Ketchup*
1 TT	*Mustard*
1 TB	*Natural yoghurt*

For the filling:

125 g	*Minced meat*
	Salt and pepper
1 disc	*Melted cheese (e.g. shaded cheese)*
2	*Sour cucumbers*
something	*Salad*
2	*Tomato(s)*

Preparation:

Working time approx. 35 min. cooking time approx. 20 min. Total time approx. 55 min.

Mix skimmed quark, grater cheese and eggs into a thick mass and spread on a baking sheet lined with baking paper. Bake in a hot oven at 180 °C over/under heat for about 20 minutes. Allow the dough to cool.

Mix the ingredients for the sauce.

Fry the minced meat in a pan with salt and pepper. Cut the cucumbers into slices and add to the minced meat.

Divide 2/3 of the sauce on the baked dough. Spread the still warm minced meat over it and melt the toast cheese over the minced meat.

Then cut the salad and possibly tomatoes and place on top, spread the remaining sauce on top. Roll the dough with the baking paper so that the prepared cheese roll looks like a biscuit roll.

Salmon dish with oven vegetables:

Ingredients for 1 serving:

125 g	Salmon fillet(s), also TK
1/2 m.-sized	Zucchini
1/2 m.-sized	Paprikaschote(s), red or yellow
150 g	Small tomatoes
75 g	Mushrooms
50 g	Sheep's cheese
1 toe/n	Garlic
something	Salt and pepper

something   Olive oil

Preparation:

Working time approx. 15 min. Cooking/baking time approx. 30 min. Total time approx. 45 min.

Let the salmon fillet, if TK, thaw a little. Wash and pat dry. Season with salt and pepper, if desired also with herbs.

Cut sheep's cheese into cubes. Cut the courgettes and mushrooms into thin slices, cut the peppers into strips. Halve or quarter tomatoes. Finely chop the garlic. Mix the vegetables with the garlic, salt and pepper and a few splashes of chilli oil in a bowl.

Form a "bowl" on a baking sheet made of aluminium foil, i.e. slap up the edges on 4 sides. I recommend taking 2 layers of aluminum foil, then nothing can leak.

Alternatively, a run-up form can be used. Then spread the vegetables on top. Then add the salmon fillet to the place, sprinkle with a little olive oil and generously crumb the sheep's cheese over it. Cook in the oven at 180 °C top/under heat, approx. 30 - 35 minutes.

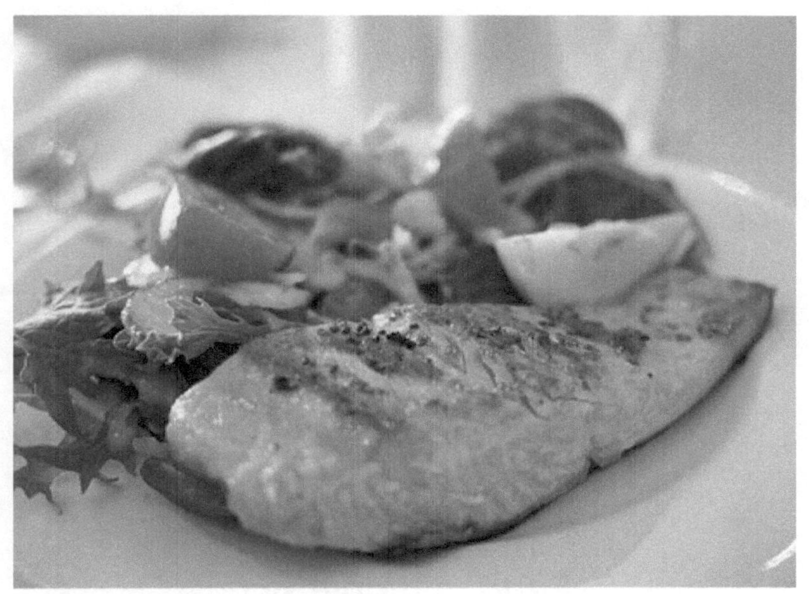

Zucchini lasagne:

Ingredients for 1 serving:

250g	*Zucchini*
125 g	*Beef mince*
50g	*Onion(s)*
¼	*Clove garlic*
100g	*Tomatoes*
50g	*Cream cheese*
25 ml	*Milk*
1 TB	*Sour*

1 TB	Tomato paste
50g	Cheese, grated
something	Olive oil
	Oregano
	Thyme
	Parsley
	Salt and pepper
	Paprika, noble sweet

Preparation:

Working time approx. 40 min. Cooking/baking time approx. 40 min. Total time approx. 80 min.

Wash zucchini and cut lengthways into finger-thick slices. Fry in a frying pan in olive oil from both sides, then drain on kitchen paper. Or sprinkle the slices with olive oil, salt a little tand brown on the top rail with the grill function in the oven. However, this takes longer.

Cut the onion into cubes and steam in the pan in a little

olive oil. Press the garlic clove and steam a little. Add the minced meat and fry crumbly. When the meat has been coloured, season with salt, pepper and paprika powder, add 1 tbsp tomato paste, stir and sweat for a minute. Add the tomatoes and season with oregano, thyme, salt, pepper and pepper. Simmer for 10 min on a small flame, then add the chopped parsley.

Mix the cream cheese with the milk, stirring either also sour cream. Season with salt, pepper and some nutmeg, stir in about 50 g of cream cheese.

Lay out a (if necessary, somewhat greased) lasagne shape or other inertia with courgettes. Spread a few spoonfuls of tomato-chopped sauce, then a layer of cream cheese sauce, and then again slices of courgettes. Continue to layer until all ingredients have been consumed. The top layer should be tomato-chopped sauce. Sprinkle with the remaining cheese and bake the zucchini lasagne in a preheated oven in about 30 minutes until golden brown.

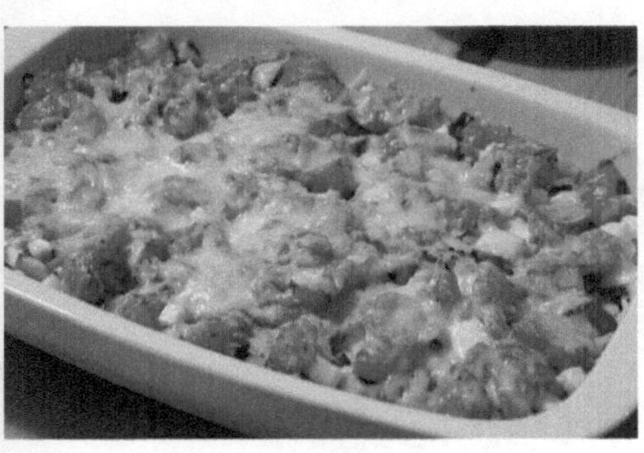

Mozzarella chicken with curry sauce:

Ingredients for 1 serving:

150g	*Chicken breast fillet(s)*
	Salt and pepper
1 TT	*Oil*
60g	*Cocktail tomatoes*
5g	*Curry powder*
30 g	*Cream*
25 g	*Cream melted cheese*
30 g	*Mozzarella*
n. B.	*Parmesan*
n. B.	*Herb*

Preparation:

Working time approx. 20 min. cooking time approx. 30 min. Total time approx. 50 min.

Wash the meat and pat dry. Season with salt and pepper. Heat the oil in a frying pan. Fry chicken breast fillet in it from all sides for about 5 minutes.

Wash and halve tomatoes. Curry powder.

Bring the cream to the boil in a saucepan. Stir in the melted cheese together with the curry powder and let it melt. Season with salt and pepper. Possibly season meat

and tomatoes with pepper

in a greased frying pan. Pour the curry cream sauce over it. Cut the mozzarella into small pieces and spread on the meat. If you like, you can spread grated parmesan and 1 tbsp herb butter into small flakes on top. Bake in a preheated oven (200 degrees or 175 degrees for circulating air) for about 30 min. Remove and optionally sprinkle with additional spices.

Tomato-mozzarella-nude run:

Ingredients for 1 serving:

100 g	Rigatoni or Penne
30g	Onion(s)
1/2 toe	Garlic
30g	Chili peppers, fresh
125 g	Tomatoes, passed

80ml	Cream
10g	Parmesan, freshly grated
30g	Mozzarella
100 g	Cherry tomato(s)
1/4 Covenant	Basil, fresh
something	Olive oil
If necessary	Salt and pepper, black

Preparation:

Working time approx. 30 min. Cooking time approx. 30 min. Total time approx. 60 min.

Preheat the oven to 200 °C (circulating air 180 °C).

Cut the onion and garlic very finely. Remove the chilli pepper and chop just as finely. Wash and halve the cherry tomatoes. Rub the parmesan and roughly dice the mozzarella. Peel the basil leaves, wash and pat dry.

Bring salted water to the boil in a large pot and cook the noodles in it, according to the package.

Meanwhile, heat olive oil in a large frying pan and sweat the onion, garlic and chilli *pepper. Add the tomatoes and simmer the sauce lightly for a few minutes. Then stir in the cream and grated parmesan and season the sauce with salt, pepper and a neat pinch of sugar.* When the noodles are ready, drain them and add to the pan to the sauce.

Remove the pan from the heat and add the halved cherry tomatoes and half of the mozzarella cubes. Cut the basil leaves into strips and also undercut them. Put *everything together in a frying pan, sprinkle with the remaining mozzarella and gratinate on the middle rail in the oven for about 20 minutes.*

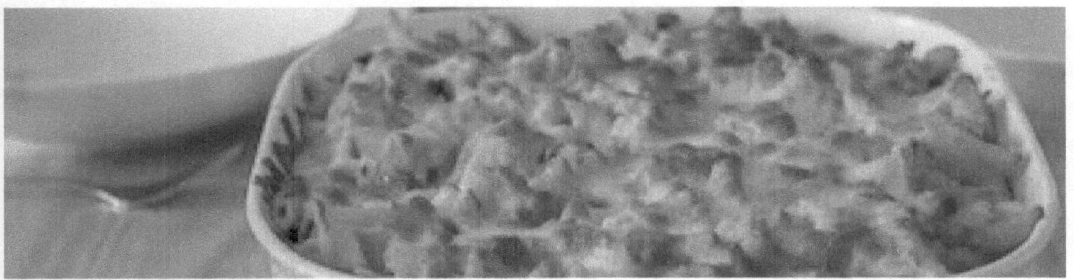

Low-carb desserts:

Chocolate quark dessert:

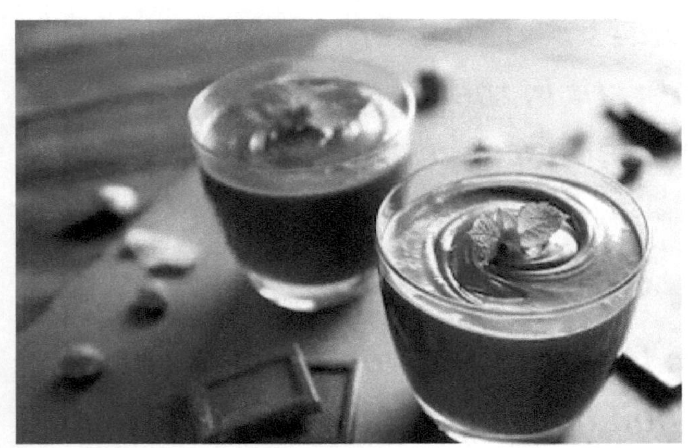

Ingredients for 1 serving:

250g	Skimmed quark
2 TB	Water
2 TB	Cocoa powder, de-oiled and unsweetened
2 TL	Sweetener, liquid, less as needed
	Vanilla or orange flavour, liquid, sugar-free

Preparation:

Working time approx. 5 min. Total time approx. 5 min.

Process skimmed quark with water, sweetener and aroma to a smooth consistency and add the cocoa. Stir everything to a homogeneous mass.

Quark dessert (like semolina porridge):

Ingredients for 1 serving:

250 g	*Cauliflower*
40g	*Cream cheese (watch out: reduced fat often reduces the taste)*
1/2 Cup	*Sweetener, (stevia or other sweetness at will)*
1/2 spoon	*Lemon zest or orange zest, finely rubbed*

Preparation:

Working time approx. 15 min. Total time approx. 15 min.

The origin of this recipe is a savoury low carb puree, which can also be prepared wonderfully sweet thanks to the relatively tasteless cauliflower. This dish is most likely to be compared to semolina porridge, but it is a very special taste and, thanks to the cream cheese, a trace of salty.

Cook the

cabbage, slightly firmer or softer depending on the desired consistency. As soon as it is cooked, puree with the cream cheese, here too, depending on the desired consistency of the pre-season, one can also use a little more or less cream cheese. Then sweeten the porridge with stevia or the desired sweetener, add the grated zest, mix well and chill the ready-made porridge.

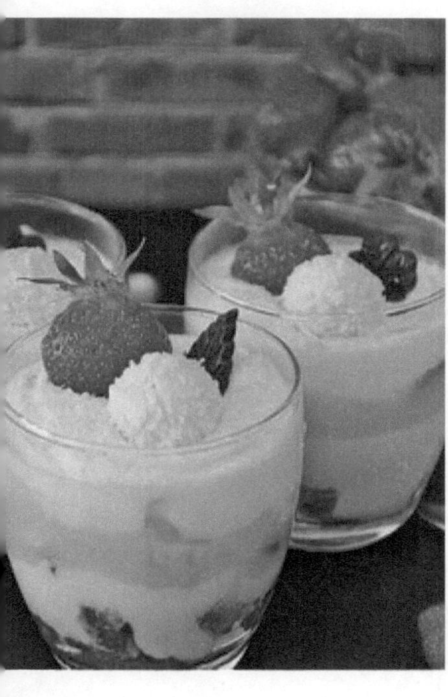

Let these recipes taste you!

*I would be very pleased to have this book reviewed.
Enjoy your life and life like a king.*

Zoe Anderleen

www.ingramcontent.com/pod-product-compliance
Lightning Source LLC
Chambersburg PA
CBHW031250250726
48655CB00005B/2155